DISCLAIMER

The information presented in this report solely and fully represents the views of the author as of the date of publication. Any omission, or potential misrepresentation of, any peoples or companies, is entirely unintentional. As a result of changing information, conditions or contexts, this author reserves the right to alter content at their sole discretion impunity.

The report is for informational purposes only and while every attempt has been made to verify the information contained herein, the author assumes no responsibility for errors, inaccuracies, and omissions. Each person has unique needs and this book cannot take these individual differences into account. For ease of use, all links in this book are redirected through this link to facilitate any future changes and minimize dead links.

TABLE OF CONTENTS

INTRODUCTION

A person who is fit is capable of living life to its fullest extent. Physical and mental fitness play very important roles in our lives and people who are both physically and mentally fit are less prone to medical conditions as well.

Fitness does not only refer to being physically fit but also refers to a person's mental state as well. If a person is physically fit, but mentally unwell or troubled, he or she will not be able to function optimally. Mental fitness can only be achieved if your body is functioning well. You can help relax your mind and eliminate stresses by exercising regularly and eating right.

People who are physically fit are also healthier, are able to maintain their most optimum weight, and are also not prone to cardiac and other health problems. To maintain a relaxed state of mind, a person should be physically active. A person who is fit both physically and mentally is strong enough to face the ups and downs of life and is not affected by drastic changes if they take place.

This book tries to point out some fitness and self-care secrets as well as strategies and rules to achieve ultimate fitness.

FITNESS

Maintaining a good level of physical fitness is something that we should all aspire to do. But it can be difficult to determine what fitness entails. Here we answer the question: what does being physically fit mean?

According to the United States Department of Health and Human Services, physical fitness is defined as "a set of attributes that people have or achieve that relates to the ability to perform physical activity."

This description goes beyond being able to run fast or lift heavy weights. Despite being important, these attributes only address single areas of fitness.

Fast facts on fitness:

- ❖ Maintaining physical fitness can help prevent some diseases.
- ❖ With exercise, body composition can change without changing weight.
- ❖ Athletes' hearts show different changes dependent on their chosen sport.
- ❖ Muscle strength increases by fiber hypertrophy and neural changes.
- ❖ Stretching to increase flexibility can ease some medical complaints.

How do you tell if someone is physically fit?

Being physically fit depends on how well a person fulfills each of the components of being healthful.

When it comes to fitness, these components include cardiorespiratory fitness, muscular strength, muscular endurance, body composition, and flexibility.

So, you can tell if someone is physically fit by determining how well they perform in each component. Here we will look at them all individually.

The Five Phases of Fitness (Psychological)

Below are the five phases we all go through when starting a new fitness program no matter what fitness level we are.

- ❖ Make a decision to get healthy; this takes 3-4 seconds, but it takes about 2-3 weeks to make a habit - hang in there at least that long and build good habits.
- ❖ You doubt yourself. It is absolutely natural to have doubts about what you are undertaking. My advice is to start doubting yourself as quickly as possible and get over it. Realize self-doubt is part of the process; even Navy SEAL trainees doubt themselves, but those who become SEALs conquer their doubt.
- ❖ Conquer Doubt - You can do anything you set your mind to. That is what you just told yourself. This is where the mind and body connect. Use the workouts to be a catalyst in all areas of your life: work, relationships, school, etc. I am a firm believer that exercising your body will give you the stamina and energy to exercise your mind and build better relationships with those around you.
- ❖ Associate yourself with fit and healthy people. By being around others who are fit, you will be inspired to also become fit in mind and body. In turn, your fitness will inspire others. Be a role model to someone trying to get in shape. People will be amazed by your new work ethic at work and play.
- ❖ Eating healthy is now a habit for you too; In fact eating lousy food makes you feel lousy.

Set and conquer a goal for yourself. Pick whatever you like - run, swim, bike, weight lift and so on – and go for it. Challenge yourself to run a 10k, swim 50 laps, lift 400 lbs, etc.

Components of Fitness

Depending on the source, the components of fitness vary considerably. Below are common components:

Cardiorespiratory Endurance

Cardiorespiratory endurance indicates how well our body can supply fuel during physical activity via the body's circulatory and respiratory systems. Activities that help improve cardiorespiratory endurance are those that cause an elevated heart rate for a sustained period.

These activities include:

- ❖ swimming
- ❖ brisk walking
- ❖ jogging
- ❖ cycling

People who regularly take part in these activities are more likely to be physically fit in terms of cardiorespiratory endurance. It is important to begin these activities slowly and gradually increase the intensity.

Exercising increases cardiorespiratory endurance in some ways. The heart muscle is strengthened so that it can pump more blood per heartbeat.

At the same time, additional small arteries are grown within muscle tissue so that blood can be delivered to working muscles more effectively when needed.

How heart health changes with exercise

The heart changes and improves its efficiency after persistent training. However, more recent research shows that different types of activity change the heart in subtly different ways.

All types of exercise increase the heart's overall size, but there are significant differences between endurance athletes, like rowers, and strength athletes, like football players. Endurance athletes' hearts show expanded left and right ventricles, whereas strength athletes show thickening of their heart wall, particularly the left ventricle.

How lung health changes with exercise

While the heart steadily strengthens over time, the respiratory system does not adjust to the same degree. Lung function does not drastically change, but oxygen that is taken in by the lungs is used more effectively.

In general, exercise encourages the body to become more efficient at taking on, distributing, and using oxygen. This improvement, over time, increases endurance and overall health.

The American College of Sports Medicine recommends aerobic exercise 3-5 times per week for 30-60 minutes, at an intensity that keeps the heart rate at 65-85 percent of the maximum heart rate.

Health benefits of Cardiorespiratory Endurance

Cardiorespiratory endurance has been found to help reduce the risk of conditions including:

- ❖ heart disease
- ❖ lung cancer
- ❖ type 2 diabetes
- ❖ stroke

Muscular strength

The U.S. Department of Health and Human Services defines muscular strength as "the ability of the muscle to exert force during an activity."

There are some ways to measure muscular strength. Lifting or pushing something of a set weight in a prescribed position and comparing the results against any given population is the best way.

In general, if a muscle is worked consistently and regularly, it will increase in strength. There are various ways of putting your muscles through rigorous activity, but anything that works a muscle until it is tired will increase muscle strength over time.

How does muscle structure change with exercise?

Muscles consist of elongated muscle cells. Each muscle cell contains contractile proteins - actin and myosin - that give the muscle its strength. These fibers contract together, producing the so-called power stroke. The total force depends on the number of these units contracting in unison.

To build muscle, the following criteria must be met:

- ❖ muscles are regularly exercised
- ❖ the individual has taken in enough protein

The exact mechanism of muscle building is not fully understood, but the general principles are well known. Training causes the muscle cells to expand, and there is an increase in actin and myosin production.

Also, in untrained muscles, fibers tend to fire asynchronously - in other words, they do not fire in unison. As they become trained, they learn to fire together as one, increasing maximum power output.

Normally, the body prevents the muscles from over-exerting themselves and becoming injured. As the muscle is trained, the body starts to disinhibit the muscles' activation - more power is allowed to be exerted.

Muscular endurance

Fitness can include muscular endurance, which is the ability of a muscle to continue exerting force without tiring. As mentioned above, strength training builds bigger muscles. Endurance training, on the other hand, does not necessarily generate muscles of a larger size.

This is because the body focuses more on the cardiovascular system, ensuring that the muscles receive the oxygenated blood they need to keep functioning. Another important change in muscles that are specifically trained for endurance concerns the different types of muscle tissue - fast twitch and slow twitch fibers:

Fasts twitch fibers

Contract quickly but get tired quickly. They use a lot of energy and are useful for sprints. They are whitish as they do not require blood to function.

Slow twitch fibers

Best for endurance work, they can carry out tasks without getting tired. They are found in core muscles. These fibers appear red as they rely on a good supply of oxygenated blood and contain stores of myoglobin.

Different exercises will promote fast twitch fibers, slow twitch fibers, or both. A sprinter will have comparatively more fast twitch fibers, whereas a long distance runner will have slower twitch fibers.

Body composition

Body composition measures the relative amounts of muscle, bone, water, and fat.

An individual can potentially maintain the same weight but radically change the ratio of each of the components that make up the body.

For instance, people with a high muscle (lean mass) ratio weigh more than those with the same height and waist circumference who have less muscle. Muscle weighs more than fat, depending on the activity that the individual is being trained to carry out.

Flexibility

Flexibility is the range of movement across a joint. Flexibility is important because it improves the ability to link movements together smoothly and can help prevent injuries. Flexibility is specific to each joint and depends on some variables, including the tightness of ligaments and tendons.

Flexibility is increased by various activities, all designed to stretch joints, ligaments, and tendons. Three types of exercise are generally utilized to increase flexibility:

Dynamic stretching

This is the ability to complete a full range of motion of a particular joint. This type of flexibility is used in standard "warming up" exercises as it helps ready the body for physical activity.

Static-active stretching

Holding the body or part of the body in a stretched position and maintaining that position for a period of time. One example of static-active stretching is the splits.

Ballistic stretching

Only to be used when the body is already warmed up and limber from exercise, it involves stretching in various positions and bouncing.

There are some ways to improve flexibility. A daily stretching regimen can be the simplest and most efficient way of achieving whole body flexibility.

Rules to Achieve Ultimate Fitness

Get out of your comfort zone

"Insanity is doing the same thing over and over again and expecting different results," said Albert Einstein. There is no need to go and spend an hour in the gym on the cross trainer. It would be like going to a museum and spending an hour in the reception. We were born to push, pull, climb and train the body in a variety of movements, so it's important to alternate between different high-intensity sculpting exercises. But it's just as important to rest hard too. Varied types of exercise stimulate the body and the brain: start every morning by dancing to get your day off to the best start. Essentially, getting out of your comfort zone is the best way to see change, as much physical as mental.

Avoid fructose before and after sport

Why? Because it slows down the fat-burning effects of a workout. Fat after a workout has also been shown to have a detrimental effect. That means no banana before or during a session as they are overly rich in sugar and the same goes for sugary energy drinks that are too often available at gyms. An overdose of sugar can be bad for your cognitive function and dramatically counteract weight-loss so instead, opt for protein and fibrous carbohydrates. The ideal snack before a workout is organic coffee, cocoa butter, and five almonds. After a workout, enjoy lean meat or fish, green vegetables, and quinoa.

Prioritize

Your priorities dictate your choices. If you want to be on top form and look your best, you might have to think about cutting out some things and working a bit harder.

Reward your efforts by eating

"Improve your life by adding things to your diet rather than removing things. It's better to say 'I will have vegetables with my meal' instead of 'I won't have any carbs with any of my meals'. Why not plan a cheat meal at the end of the week as a way of indulging yourself without losing sight of your goals? Don't let someone make you feel guilty for having a slice of cake; whatever makes you happy is all that matters. We're only human, and you will crave foods and occasionally have lapses. It's important not to beat yourself up if you have a dessert while eating out now and then. It's not going to hurt you.

Go for a walk after a meal

Going for a brisk 10 to 30-minute walk after a meal is enough to increase the body's ability to deal with blood sugar and what's more, it can reduce the chance of diabetes.

Prepare your breakfast before going to sleep

Decide on your breakfast before bed. Most people blame a lack of time for not eating a good breakfast, but that's not an excuse to go hungry. If your mornings are busy, use leftovers from the night before and simply reheat. Try to use protein powders, eggs, salmon or pre-cooked meats. The key is high protein and good fats.

Have a quick 10-20 minute nap

Nothing is better for increasing the body's energy levels and vitality. Sleep restores the body and mind better than anything else. Research shows that taking naps of between 10-20 minutes can have a very beneficial, restorative effect on the body and mind - making it the ultimate way to create energy. Plus it has no negative side effects.

Add super nutritious ingredients to your diet

What do the following things all have in common: Fermented vegetables such as sauerkraut, kombucha, kefir, cultured butter, aloe vera, L-glutamine supplements, fiber, bone broth, cucumber and pro-biotics (ideally containing 3-5 billion live microorganisms and different strands of bacteria)? The common denominator for these is that they are all packed with nutrients that have a wonderful effect on fitness and well-being.

Make your goals visible

Once you've organized your goals, put them on your mirror or fridge or anywhere where you'll constantly be reminded of them. You can always start over if you lose your focus.

Sleep more

This is the number one rule. After working out, I make sure I have good quality sleep. It's an essential moment of relaxation where the body recuperates after exercise and repairs torn muscle tissue. A lack of sleep increases cortisol levels, a hormone that undos the benefits of exercise and suppresses fat burning, not to mention the increased hunger pangs that it stimulates. If you can't sleep, check your magnesium levels as a deficiency could be to blame. Ideally, go to bed at 10 pm as often as possible. The old adage, "Early to bed, and early to rise makes a man healthy, wealthy and wise." couldn't be truer!

Stay in the present moment

Be in 'the now' as much as you can. Make sure your breathing is full and deep; it's the best detox possible. Anything can be a moment of meditation, whether it's walking, yoga, or taking out the bins. Turn off your television and read more, spend less time on your phone, only answer your emails once a day and limit social media. These things get in the way of real life, and you get lost in a strange world based on peer pressure and competitive boasting. My advice is to live in the present moment, hold eye contact during a conversation and get out into nature as often as possible.

Love yourself unconditionally

Or you can never love anyone else unconditionally. Judgment is so boring; Don't judge and don't take anything personally. Do not underestimate yourself and overestimate others; you are stronger than you think. Plus, remember that 99 per cent of the things that you're worried about are made-up scenarios in your head that will never manifest. Wake up, take a deep breath, and be thankful to be healthy and alive.

CALISTHENICS

Do You Have Time to Exercise??

Do you really not have enough time in your day to exercise? Too many times people say, "I need to exercise, but I do not have enough time in the day." Or, when they do have the time they only have the energy to lie down and watch TV.

Exercise is anything other than sleeping or sitting. Even when you are on the floor flat on your back or stomach, you can exercise the torso with abdominal exercise or the back with other torso exercises. The push up is a great "laying down" exercise, and an abdominal crunch is just a little bit harder than resting. An hour a day is a nice goal to achieve to increase your fitness level and overall health, but even 10-15 minutes is better than nothing and beneficial too.

Fitting fitness into a day is a challenge we all face. Exercising is tough after long hours of working at home, the office or on the road, but Americans still need to work out as we are creating a generation of people who are obese and have other preventable health disorders. Many people who struggle to fit fitness into their schedule actually do a better job at getting the job done If they take 15-20 minutes before starting work for the day and 15-20 minutes after work is done for the day. Even if that exercise is a simple walk before breakfast and after dinner, a 15-20 minute walk at each of these times can significantly help you burn calories that may have ended up being stored as fat otherwise. In fact, after any meal, a light walk and some calisthenics will help you to be more energized and ready to do whatever.

Why Bodyweight Training?

Changing people's minds about certain things can be hard. And one of them, I've found, is preconceived notions about different fitness methods. A lot of people think the definition of fitness is the inflated bodybuilder like we've all seen in fitness magazines. That's never been my fitness goal, and I think I'm a better athlete for it. But it can be really tough to convince people that bodyweight training is a viable option for getting in shape.

They can be done anywhere. I know I've already mentioned this, but it bears repeating. This is perfect for beginners that may be self-conscious about starting out. With bodyweight training, there's no obligation to work out in a giant, crowded building with strangers. It can just be you, an open space in your living room, and your pets (and you know they'd never judge you!). And when you're traveling; either for work or fun, calisthenics is a great way to avoid losing progress when you're away from home. So you can vacation with confidence, knowing that you can take your workout routine along with you!

It's a big time saver. Before I got into calisthenics, if you had asked me how long people need to spend in the gym to get in shape, I would have said an hour a day at least. This idea is not only false; it's counter-productive to the progression of fitness. People are busy enough, and if you tell them they have to set aside over an hour a day to get in shape, they'll be discouraged before they even begin! So they don't even give fitness a shot, and their health suffers. I'm here to show you that you can get a great workout in a fraction of the time by using time optimization workouts. That's what I'm presenting you with today.

No heavy equipment is required. Something else I've already talked about, but I thought I'd say it again, just in case there was anyone out there with their credit card in hand, ready to order the newest exercise gizmo being advertised on TV right now; Put the card down and step away slowly. You already have the tools you need to get in shape. Sure, calisthenics utilizes a few tools to optimize a workout or target a specific area.

It builds solid, lean muscle. This is the one where people tend to tilt their heads and look at me funny. That's alright; I'm used to it. The fact is, most people think if you want to build solid muscle, you have to lift heavy weights. It's simply not true, and I'm living proof of that. The great thing about calisthenics is it forces your body to act as a unit. Think about the sitting dumbbell curl exercise. The only muscle group being targeted is the bicep. Every other part of your body is just sitting there, wondering when they're going to get a turn to exercise. With calisthenics, your body acts as a chain: one muscle group must utilize others in order to execute the exercise or maneuver, and as a result, you're going to build solid, lean muscle much faster.

It's great for fat loss. Calisthenics can be a great cardiovascular tool. Now, by that, I don't mean I'm going to send you jogging for ten miles a day. You can get an outstanding cardio workout without countless laps around your block. There are plenty of programs (including the one you're about to see) that, if done correctly, can be a great method for fat loss.

It improves mobility. There are some complicated exercises in the world of bodyweight training! You'll see that even with this beginner program. But learning them will dramatically improve your balance, flexibility and overall mobility. That's because as your body relies on a number of different muscle groups to perform an exercise, you're going to be training your body to act as a unit without you even knowing it!

Exercise and Healthy Eating is the First Priority

An exercise program aims to lose fat without losing muscle and without reducing metabolic rate. The exercise needs to be customized to fitness level and specific goal of fat loss.

Together, aerobic exercise and resistance training are the ideal combinations of exercise to achieve fat loss, and they should be part of your lifestyle.

Aerobic Exercise

Aerobic exercise metabolizes calories and raises the metabolic rate. The heart rate needs to be raised to a certain level for 20 - 30 minutes at least three times per week. By exercising aerobically, calories will be burnt at a rate of 300+ per hour depending on your weight and fitness level.

If you consider that just 1 pound of body fat has approximately 4,100 calories, then you can get a rough idea of just how long it will take to shed those extra pounds permanently. Think of how long it took to put on those pounds, so it will also take time to take off those same pounds.

Personally, I recommend that you work at a level that you know that you can maintain for a minimum of 20 to 30 minutes. The debate comes in, when various fitness bodies suggest training at a high heart rate of 75/90% of max, for short periods or at 55/80% of maximum heart rate for easier, longer periods.

In short try both methods, unless you are a complete beginner to fitness, in which case I would recommend training at a steady pace for as long as comfortably possible.

Aerobic exercise will also raise the metabolic rate for approximately 24 hours after you have finished training. This helps to burn up extra calories and prevents the metabolic rate from declining.

Resistance (or weight) Training

Inactive people lose about 10% of their muscle mass every ten years after the age of 25. However, with regular resistance training, it is possible to regain this muscle mass.

Resistance training should be carried out 2-3 times per week for approximately 30 minutes. Although not generally effective as aerobic training for burning calories, resistance training will still burn about 250-500 calories per hour and will raise the metabolic rate.

Weight training will not develop your body to resemble a body builder, but it will create the ability to burn more calories in a 24 hour period. Another important point is that muscle will not turn into fat, if you stop training. The muscle tissue will naturally break down and shrink in size.

An important point to remember is that lean muscle tissue weighs more than body fat, so your actual body weight may stay the same during the early stages of your new lifestyle regime.

Don't be alarmed; the weight will come off. However, if it does not, your overall ratio of body fat compared to lean muscle tissue will certainly be in a healthier ratio.

Try and avoid using the scale for this reason, unless it can monitor your body fat as well. Instead measure your body at various points, e.g., your hips, chest, stomach, and thighs. Using an item of clothing is also a good way to measure yourself, as with a bit of time and dedication, you will find that the clothing fits you properly. You will, at a point, lose inches but stop losing weight for about a 2-4 week period typically.

Getting Started

The following stretching plan will assist you with getting started again safely and without as much post-exercise soreness.

Too many people above the age of 30 get injured no matter what they are doing. From shoveling snow, a pickup basketball game and simply walking across a parking lot in winter, most injuries are strains or muscle pulls that can be prevented with a few simple stretching exercises done daily. The added flexibility will not only assist in injury prevention, but with speed workouts, will better enable you to run faster. The following is a stretching routine that can be used whether you are a beginner or advanced athlete.

The Television Workout Option:

Did you know that there are 10 minutes of commercials for every 30 minute TV show? If you watch TV for an hour and exercise during the commercials, you can actually engage in 20 minutes of metabolism charging exercise.

The Stretching Program

Increasing one's flexibility should be the first goal before starting a fitness program. In fact, if you are thinking about beginning a fitness program and you have been idle for many years, you should stretch for an entire week before you start running, lifting weights, or doing any calisthenics exercise. It is alright to walk to warm up, however.

So, your first 1-2 weeks of starting a fitness program should consist of the following stretches 1-2 times a day, drinking 2-3 liters of water a day, and walking, biking or some other non-impact, low-intensity cardio activity for 10-15 minutes.

Hold these stretches or do these movements for at least 15-20 seconds each:

- ❖ Shoulder Shrugs
- ❖ Chest / Bicep Stretch
- ❖ Arm/Shoulder Stretch
- ❖ Triceps/Back Stretch (half moon)
- ❖ Stomach Stretch
- ❖ Lower back Stretch
- ❖ ITB / Hip
- ❖ Calf Stretch
- ❖ Hamstring Stretch
- ❖ Thigh Stretch - standing or laying on floor

Stretch in this order to aid in major muscle group stretching. Stretching the connecting groups of the thighs and hamstrings first will assist in a more thorough stretch of the hams and thighs – the major muscle groups of the body.

Stretching and Warming Up

Holding these stretches for 15-20 seconds is the best way to begin your workout. Do not bounce when performing these stretches and inhale deeply for three seconds, hold for three seconds and fully exhale. Do this twice per stretch. This will take you to the 15-20 second time minimum for holding these stretches for optimal results.

Explanations of the Stretches

Arm / Shoulder Circles - Rotate your shoulders slowly in big circles forward and reverse for 15 seconds in each direction and as if you were swimming the backstroke and front crawl stroke.

Chest / Shoulder / Upper Back Stretch

Grab onto a pole or wall and twist opposite of your arm until you feel the stretch in your chest and shoulder connection. Repeat with the other arm. Option two; the swimmer stretch: If you can, grasp your hands behind your back and pull your shoulders back standing upright with your chest out. Then roll the shoulders forward and place your chin to your chest.

Arm Shoulder Stretch

Grab your arm with the opposite arm and pull it across the body stretching the rear shoulder and upper back. Rotate hands with thumbs down.

Shoulder Rotations

This movement helps warm up the rotator cuff of the shoulder joint and is a great one to do if you are about the throw a ball or just need to work on full range of motion of the shoulder.

Torso Twists

Stay in the same position but now twist to the left and right trying to keep your hips facing forward.

Triceps into Back Stretch

Place both arms over and behind your head. Grab your right elbow with your left hand and pull your elbow toward your opposite shoulder. Lean with the pull; Repeat with the other arm.

Abdominal Stretch

Lie on your stomach. Push yourself up to your elbows. Slowly lift your head and shoulders and look up at the sky or ceiling. Hold for 15 seconds and repeat two times.

Lower back Stretch #1 Cat Stretch

Try to hold your head as close to your shoulders as possible. Put your chin to your chest and hold for 10 seconds.

Lower back Stretch #2 Lie on your left side

Place your top leg in front of you. Slowly twist your torso until your shoulders touch the floor. Hold for 15 seconds and repeat on the right side.

As you may know, the lower back is the most commonly injured area of the body. Many lower back problems stem from inactivity, lack of flexibility, and improper lifting of heavy objects. Stretching and exercising your lower back will help prevent some of those injuries.

Calf Stretch into Achilles Tendon Stretch

Stand with one foot 2-3 feet in front of the other. With both feet pointing in the same direction as you are facing, put most of your body weight on your leg that is behind you – stretching the calf muscle.

Now, bend the rear knee slightly. You should now feel the stretch in your heel. This stretch helps prevent Achilles tendonitis, a severe injury that will sideline most people for about 4-6 weeks.

Down Dog Pose

1. Begin on your hands and knees. Align your wrists directly under your shoulders and your knees directly under your hips. Point your middle fingers directly to the top edge of your mat.

2. Stretch your elbows and relax your upper back.

3. Spread your fingers wide and press firmly through your palms and knuckles. Distribute your weight evenly across your hands.

4. Exhale as you tuck your toes and lift your knees off the floor. Reach your pelvis up toward the ceiling, then draw your buttock bones toward the wall behind you. Gently begin to straighten your legs, but do not lock your knees. Bring your body into the shape of an "A." Imagine your hips and

thighs being pulled backwards from the top of your thighs. Do not walk your feet closer to your hands — keep the extension of your whole body.

5. Press the floor away from you as you lift through your pelvis. As you lengthen your spine, lift your buttock bones up toward the ceiling. Now press down equally through your heels and the palms of your hands.

6. Tighten the outer muscles of your arms and press your index fingers into the floor. Lift from the inner muscles of your arms to the top of both shoulders. Draw your shoulder blades into your upper back ribs and toward your tailbone. Broaden across your collarbones.

7. Rotate your arms externally so your elbow creases face your thumbs.

8. Draw your chest toward your thighs as you continue to press the mat away from you, lengthening and decompressing your spine.

9. Engage your quadriceps. Rotate your thighs inward as you continue to lift your buttock bones high. Sink your heels toward the floor.

10. Align your ears with your upper arms. Relax your head, but do not let it dangle. Gaze between your legs or toward your navel.

11. Hold for 5-100 breaths.

12. To release, exhale as you gently bend your knees and come back to your hands and knees.

Hamstring Stretch

From the standing or sitting position, bend forward at the waist and touch your toes. Keep your back straight and slightly bend your knees. You should feel this stretching the back of your thighs.

Thigh Stretch Standing

While standing, bend your knee and grab your foot at the ankle. Pull your heel to your butt and push your hips forward. Squeeze your butt cheeks together and keep your knees close together. Hold for 10-15 seconds and repeat with the other leg. You can hold onto something for balance if you need to OR you can lie down on your hip and perform this stretch.

Tender Shin Exercises

If you get shin splints from running or walking, here are two great exercises to build up your shins. Stand on your heels for 10-15 seconds. Repeat a few times and even throughout the day to build up your shin muscles. Before walking and running, do the foot flex/stretch exercise 30-40 times on each leg.

Regular and Knee Push-ups

Lie on the ground with your hands placed flat next to your chest. Your hands should be about shoulder width apart. Push yourself up by straightening your arms and keeping your back stiff. This exercise will build and firm your shoulders, arms, and chest. Use your knees if necessary to complete the repetitions in the workout.

Assisted Push-ups

Using a piece of furniture to place your hands 3-4 feet off the ground; lean into the furniture or wall. Straighten your arms, back, hips, and legs and push yourself off of the firmly placed piece of furniture. Bend your arms so that your chest touches the furniture. Repeat as required. This is a great way to start out if you cannot do any push-ups at all.

Bench Dips

Sit on a chair, bench or small table. Place your feet about three feet in front of you as you sit on the very edge of the seat. Now, grab the edge of the seat with your hands, lift your butt off the seat and lower yourself about 4-5 inches below the seat by bending your arms at the elbow.

Lower Body Exercises

Squats

Keep your feet shoulder width apart. Drop your butt back as though sitting in a chair. Concentrate on squeezing your glutes in your upward motion. Keep your heels on the ground and your shins should be near vertical at all times. Extend your buttocks backward. Do not keep your buttocks over your feet and extend your knees over your feet.

The 1/2 Squat

Intensify your squat by doing 1/2 squats. While in the full squat position, hold the pose and push yourself up and down within a 6" range of motion....just like riding a horse.

Walking Squats

This is a regular squat, but you add a side hop to it. Squat down in a full squat position. When pushing yourself upward, shuffle your feet to the left or right. Each step, stop and do a full squat. You can alternate left and right steps if you do not have much room or you can do ten side squats to the left across a room then ten side squats to the right back to your starting place.

Walking Lunge

The lunge is a great leg exercise to develop shape and flexibility. Keep your chest up high and your stomach tight. Take a long step forward and drop your back knee toward the ground. Stand up on your forward leg; bringing your feet together and repeat with the other leg. Make sure your knee never extends past your foot. Keep your shin vertical in other words. Muscles used: quadriceps, hams, and glutes.

Stationary Lunge

Take a big stride forward. Bend both knees as you lower yourself, so your front thigh is near parallel to the floor. Lift yourself up, so your knees are straight, but your feet have remained in the same position. If you have bad knees either avoid the lunge exercise or only go half way down.

Abdominals

When you exercise your stomach muscles, make sure to exercise and stretch your back also. The stomach and lower back muscles are opposing muscle groups, and if one is much stronger than the other, then you can injure the weaker muscle group easily - usually the lower back.

Regular Crunch

Lie on your back with your feet and knees in the air with the knees bent. Cross your hands over your chest and bring your elbows to your knees by flexing your stomach. Keep your feet on the floor if your lower back is weak or previously injured.

Reverse Crunch

In the same position as the regular crunch, lift your knees and butt toward your elbows. Leave your head and upper body flat on the ground. Only move your legs and butt.

Right Elbow to Left Knee

Cross your left leg over your right leg. Flex your stomach and twist to bring your right elbow to your left knee.

Left Elbow to Right Knee

Cross your right leg over your leg. Flex your stomach and twist to bring your left elbow to your right knee.

Double Crunch - (Legs up)

Lie on your back with your feet in the air. Cross your hands over your chest and bring your elbows to your knees by flexing your stomach and lift your hips off the floor as if you were doing a reverse crunch. This is a two crunches in one movement (do not do if you have previous lower back injury).

Bicycle Crunches – (Love handles)

Peddle your legs back and forth while doing left and right crunches. This is a tough one, so if your back hurts, stop and save this exercise until your back is stronger.

Lower Back Exercises

These exercises are to be done immediately following any large set of abdominals in order to balance out the torso with the opposing muscle group of the abdominals / lower back. You will find that a strong lower back will assist you in completing long, load bearing hikes.

Plank Pose

Do not allow your hips and butt to sag too low or poke up too high — it's important to keep your body in one straight line, from shoulders to heels. Keep your shoulders aligned directly over your wrists. The distance between your hands and feet should be the same.

Prone Lower Back Exercise #1

Lie on your stomach with your arms extended over your head. Lift your right arm and your left leg off the ground at the same time and repeat for a specified number of repetitions. Switch arms/legs and repeat.

Upper Back Exercise - (reverse pushups)

Lie on your stomach in the down push up position. Lift your hands off the floor 2-3 inches instead of pushing off the floor. This will strengthen your upper back muscles that oppose the chest muscles.

Upper Back Exercise #3 – (Birds)

Lie on your stomach with your arms spread to the height of your shoulders. Lift both arms off the floor until your shoulder blades "pinch" and place them slowly in the down position. Repeat for 10-15 repetitions mimicking a bird flying.

Lateral Raise

A safe and effective shoulder exercise with light weights or no weights as well. Using dumbbells weighing over 5 pounds is not recommended for this exercise. Keep your knees slightly bent, shoulder back, and your chest high. Lift weights parallel to ground in a smooth, controlled motion, keep your palms facing the ground. Follow the next six exercises without stopping.

Thumbs Up

After performing ten regular lateral raises, do ten lateral raises with your thumbs up, touching your hips with your palms facing away from you and raising your arms no higher than shoulder height.

Thumbs Up / Down

Continue with side lateral raises. As you lift your arms upward, keep your thumbs up. Once your arms are shoulder height, turn your hands and make your thumbs point toward the floor. Repeat for ten times, always leading in the up and down direction with your thumbs.

Front Raise (Thumbs Up)

Now, for ten more repetitions, time to work your front deltoids. Lift the dumbbells from your waist to shoulder height keeping your thumbs up.

Cross Overs

With your palms facing away from you and arms relaxed in front of your hips, bring your arms up and over your head as if you were doing a jumping jack (without jumping). Cross your arms in front of your head and bring them back to your hips for ten repetitions.

Military Press

Place one foot ahead of the other, and knees slightly bent to reduce strain on your lower back. Exhale as you push the weights over your head for ten final repetitions in this mega-shoulder pump workout. Slowly lower them to shoulder height and repeat. Muscles used are shoulders and triceps (back of arm).

Dumbbell Exercises

Biceps Curls

Stand up straight with a dumbbell in each hand at arm's length. Keep your elbows close to your torso and rotate the palms of your hands until they are facing forward. This will be your starting position. Now, keeping the upper arms stationary, exhale and curl the weights while contracting your biceps.

Hammer Curls

This is the same as bicep curls except your palms are facing your hips. Alternate lifting each dumbbell like you were running - "hip to the lip." Use a complete range of motion and keep it smooth. Do not swing the weights.

Triceps Extensions - (Back of the arm)

With weights in hands, bring your hands overhead and lower the weight toward the back of your neck. Make certain your elbows remain in one place throughout the movement – next to your ears! Repeat!

SELF-CARE SECRETS

Self-care is an essential part of balancing out an overwhelmed, stressed out lifestyle. It gives us a chance to rest and recover from the wear and tear of normal life events, and it's also a good reason to bring more fun into our lives. Sometimes we wish that others would take care of us, but the reality is that if we're not taking good care of ourselves, then we can't expect anyone else to do it for us.

It Doesn't Have To Cost Much (Or Any) Money

Of course, the ultimate self-care dream involves a week at a spa that has 5-star accommodations, all kinds of fancy facials, massages, and beauty treatments, and delicious, healthy meals prepared for us. However, the reality is that we don't have to put self-care on the back-burner until we can afford to do that. There are lots of self-care activities that you can do that cost little or no money and include at-home facials and manicures, hot bubble baths, meditation breaks throughout the day, and taking a long walk in a park on a beautiful day. Sometimes we just need to remember to make the most of our resources.

It Needs To Happen On A Regular Basis

Self-care shouldn't be an "I'll do that when I have some extra time" activity. It needs to be a "this is going to be scheduled into my calendar regularly" activity. By doing self-care activities regularly, it'll become a healthy habit and will result in decreased stress levels! If it's a sporadic thing that only happens once in a while, then your stress levels will continue to be high in between because you aren't giving yourself enough attention and relaxation time.

It Doesn't Need To Take A Lot Of Time

When you regularly keep up with your self-care, it doesn't require a lot of time. Of course, if you have a lot of time to dedicate to yourself, go for it! But the reality is we are all juggling a lot of activities and responsibilities and just dedicating a few minutes each day to caring for yourself will have positive effects on your mood. There are several self-care activities that you can do with just a few minutes, and that includes a 5-minute meditation, a 15-minute nap in the middle of the afternoon, a 10-minute massage at your local nail place, and a tea break in the middle of the work day.

It Does Require You To Be Present

In order to get the best benefits from your self-care routine, make sure you stay in the present moment while doing it. That means no stressing about the bad day you had at work or worrying about all the things that you still need to do before the end of the day. While you're doing your self-care, remember that you are deserving of this time and don't let yourself feel any guilt about what you think you "should" be doing instead. You may be going for a run, taking a yoga class, using your fancy shower gel, or just enjoying a yummy-scented candle, but keep the intention that you are doing something good for yourself because you deserve it and that's all you need to focus on at that moment.

It Doesn't Need To Be A Solo Activity

I always used to think that self-care required me to be alone while I do it because it wouldn't count as self-care if someone else was there. I now realize that's not true, and that self-care can be you spending time with your family and friends enjoying their company. Just being in the present moment with them and doing something fun is one of my favorite ways to take care of myself – it might be a day at the beach, or a weekend away, or maybe even dinner out with them. As long as you are enjoying yourself and taking time out of your hectic lifestyle, then you can count it as some self-care.

Self-Care Approaches

Personal happiness and well-being can be derived from various sources, whether it is a hobby, quality time with family or a significant other, or a rewarding volunteer commitment. This guide is designed to get you started in the right direction, but you should not limit your self-care efforts to the suggestions in this guide.

Nutrition

A healthy diet is one that provides enough of each essential nutrient, contains a variety of foods from all of the basic food groups, provides adequate energy, and does not contain excess fat, sugar, and salt.

There are many reasons to maintain a healthy diet. These include:

- ❖ Improved health
- ❖ Increased energy
- ❖ Managing weight gain
- ❖ Preventing and managing diseases and disorders

Even though eating healthy food can make us feel better, it is not always easy. Sometimes it seems much easier to grab a quick meal at a fast food restaurant instead of packing a healthy lunch at home. It can also be hard to say no when your coworkers are indulging in unhealthy snacks. It is important to remember that even little changes in diet can make a difference and big changes can make a big difference.

Below are steps you can take to improve your diet

Don't Get Overwhelmed

There are literally thousands of diets and approaches to weight loss, just look on the Best Sellers list or a magazine rack, and you will be confronted with 10 to 20 of the latest diets. Before starting a diet, be sure to research your options and consider discussing it with your physician. Consider various aspects of the diet, such as whether it will require you to prepare special foods in addition to the food you prepare for your family and the cost of the food the diet recommends. Also, the length of time you will be on a diet is a consideration. Consider whether you will stick to the diet for 30 days, 3 months, or 6 months. If the diet is not right for your lifestyle, it can be very hard to maintain.

Consider What You Are Eating

Get in the habit of reading labels and looking at the nutritional information on packages. Many restaurants also make nutritional information available. Knowing what you are eating can help you make healthy choices.

Portion Size

In addition to watching what you eat, you need to watch how much you eat. America's obesity epidemic has been attributed not only to what we are eating but how much we are eating. United States Department of Agriculture (USDA) statistics indicate that the total daily caloric intake for Americans has risen from 1,854 to 2,002 calories over the last 20 years. This increase, 148 calories per day, works out to an extra 15 pounds every year (DHHS/USDA, 2005). Techniques for limiting portion size include weighing your food, checking the serving sizes on packages, and avoiding "Super Sizing."

Plan to Eat Right

Eating right doesn't just happen, you need to plan for it. This can take the form of taking your lunch to work or having healthy snacks, such as fruits, carrot sticks, or nuts, at your desk so you can avoid the temptation of buying a candy bar or soda. If you are going to an event where you know there will be unhealthy food, have a healthy snack before you arrive. It is much easier to resist temptation if you are not hungry.

Don't Forget Water

Keeping the body well hydrated can have a significant impact on health. Almost two-thirds of our body weight is water. Water is necessary to digest food and absorb vitamins and nutrients. It plays a role in detoxifying the liver and kidneys and removing waste and toxins from the body. If you are dehydrated, the body must work harder to circulate the blood, leaving you less energy to do the things you want and need to do.

How much water should you drink? The general rule is eight 8-ounce glasses of water a day. Another way to determine how many ounces of water you should drink a day is to divide your weight by two. For example, if you weigh 150 pounds you should drink 75 ounces of water a day (150 divided by two is 75).

Tips for Staying Hydrated

- ❖ Avoid drinking liquids such as coffee, tea, or soda, which often contain caffeine. These can actually result in the loss of water from the body since caffeine is a diuretic.
- ❖ When you are exercising remember to drink plenty of water before, during, and after to compensate for the water that you may lose through perspiration.
- ❖ Drink before you feel thirsty. You are already dehydrated when you feel thirsty.
- ❖ Keep a bottle of water with you at all times.
- ❖ Make water available in places where you spend a significant amount of your time, like work. Consider setting up a water club at the office and sharing the cost of having bottled water delivered.

Recruit Others to Eat Healthily

It is much easier to eat healthy foods if others around you are doing the same. Consider recruiting a friend or co-worker and motivate each other to make healthy nutritional choices. Encourage your employer to provide healthy snacks at meetings and work-related functions (or at least some healthy alternatives).

Setting Strong Personal Standards and Boundaries

Another way to practice self-care is to learn to set strong personal standards and boundaries. Standards are those things you hold yourself to while boundaries are those things that you hold others to. Example: if you refuse to use illegal substances on principle, that's a standard. If you refuse to allow others to use illegal substances in your home or your presence, that's a boundary. High standards and clear boundaries are essential parts of self-care.

While property boundaries are marked on maps and staked out by surveyors, personal boundaries are not immediately evident to others. Personal boundaries are more like imaginary lines created to protect a person's body, mind, and spirit from the unhealthy or damaging behavior of others. Such lines are not intended to shut people out; they are designed to keep unwanted behaviors from intruding on and negatively affecting your well-being. Setting strong personal boundaries is essential for personal health and allows you to protect and take care of yourself.

The first step in setting boundaries is to identify those behaviors of others that are not acceptable to you. For example, most people have a boundary that others may not hit them. Other examples of boundaries are:

- ❖ Others may not yell at me.
- ❖ Others may not speak to me rudely.
- ❖ Others may not enter my office without knocking.
- ❖ Others may not call me at home to discuss office matters.
- ❖ Others may not gossip in my presence.

Once you have identified the behaviors that you will not tolerate, it's important to communicate your boundaries to others. People will not know what you expect from them unless you teach them how to act in your presence. Be direct when you assert your boundaries and expect that it will take several requests before others "get" that you are serious about enforcing your boundaries.

Steps To Enforcing Boundaries

- ❖ Inform by pointing out the behavior that is unacceptable: "Do you realize that you are speaking to me in an extremely loud voice?"
- ❖ Request to let the other person know what you expect: "Please do not speak to me in such a loud voice."
- ❖ Give the warning to let the person know what you will do if they continue with the unacceptable behavior: "If you continue to speak to me in such a loud voice, I will leave the room."
- ❖ Follow through with the stated consequence. It is crucial that you follow through with the consequence if the person ignores the warning: "What you are doing is unacceptable to me, so I am leaving the room. You may

come and find me when you are ready to discuss this without speaking in such a loud voice."
* Let go of the outcome. Another person's offensive behavior is not about you, even though it may feel personal.

Asking and expecting others to treat you appropriately is a necessary step in learning to take care of yourself and allows you to develop healthy relationships, exhibit self-respect, and become a role model for others.

Preventing Burnout

Burnout is a stress syndrome that is prevalent among those working in health and helping professions. It happens when people try to reach unrealistic goals and end up depleting their energy and losing touch with themselves and others in the process.

According to psychologist Herbert J. Freudenberger, Ph.D., who coined the term, burnout is "the extinction of motivation or incentive, especially where one's devotion to a cause or relationship fails to produce the desired results" (1980). Since burnout is a condition caused by good intentions, it is easy to see how preventing it is very important for coaches, bosses, and parents.

IMPORTANT: Watch for the signs and symptoms of burnout in yourself, as well as to recognizing them in other people. However, keep in mind that each person is different in how s/he exhibits and responds to burnout.

Signs of burnout can include:

* Emotions such as anger, frustration, depression
* Impatience
* Feeling tired, fatigue
* Melancholy
* Ambivalence
* Lack of interest
* Short term memory loss
* Dreading an event

- ❖ Anxiety or panic
- ❖ Self-medication
- ❖ Nightmares
- ❖ Health issues
- ❖ Difficulty making decisions
- ❖ Working at 120%, then dropping to nothing
- ❖ Not caring

Burnout prevention strategies may include:

- ❖ Know yourself – watch for your particular signs of burnout and develop strategies for relief.
- ❖ Have a support system – engage friends, family, and others to help you avoid or manage burnout.
- ❖ Maintain a calendar that works for your lifestyle – make sure that you book time and activities that recharge your batteries.
- ❖ Set and maintain boundaries following the above guidelines.
- ❖ Follow your wellness program – it's not about perfection but building in activities and choices that minimize burnout or enable a quick recovery.
- ❖ Take time off (vacations, moments, hours) to recover.
- ❖ Get 15 minutes of sunshine each day.
- ❖ Home office tricks – taking breaks, scheduling time out of the office, socialize, meet with colleagues, network. Practice ten daily habits that give you pleasure.

Let's just admit it. Every single person today wants to look and feel good.

We're more calm, present, and confident when we perform regular self-care and physical exercise. We're in tune with our needs and how to fulfill them, which encourages us to take care of ourselves so we can show up to life in a way we're proud of. This isn't about being perfect. It's about nurturing and loving yourself, so you can feel in tune with who you are and how you want to interact with the world. Prioritize little acts of fitness and self-care and feel refreshed, revived, and ready to take on whatever challenges come your way.

""Thank you for reading! I hope this book helps you. If you have a moment, please leave a review."